by the same author

My Medicine Garden
My Happy Garden
The Garden Series

The Diabetes Diary

herbalYODA Says!

Wild Medicine

**The Road to Health
Natural Care Series:**

Blood Pressure Care Naturally

By Gayle Eversole, DHom, PhD, MH, NP, ND

BLOOD PRESSURE CARE NATURALLY

Jere Goyan, MD, the authoritarian FDA Commissioner from 1979 to 1981, was quoted in the Detroit Free Press on November 5, 2003 as stating:

"We as patients have got to raise the questions ourselves and take care of our own selves."

This book is a guide to help you begin traveling on your "Road to Health". The program you develop should meet your needs and not those of another person. We are all unique and our natural health care plan should be too.

What You'll Find Inside

Acknowledgments

This book would not have come about without the support of the friends who encouraged me. My thanks go to especially Mark and Jennifer in Moscow, Idaho. For on-going encouragement from those who kept me forging ahead I thank: Dee in Lewiston, Idaho; Bonetstasia, my artistic consultant and long-time friend from Fabrications Textiles in Omaha, Nebraska; Margo, an OMD in Coeur d'Alene; Marc in New York City; James in Edmonds, Washington for being my writing coach and friend; and instructors and classmates in the fiction writing class I took for fun.

I can't overlook the patience of my animal companions who stood up under weeks of paper shuffling as I went through years of notes and files to select the information presented here.

And the friends who listened to me rant when I had to wait for months to get the copyright certificate, the times when the electronic wonder called 'my computer' froze and freshly edited files went who knew where.

I also appreciate Mike and his crew from Copy Court for their fine help with the first print run.

Most of all this project is dedicated to the many clients and friends who have helped me over the years through their gracious gift: selecting me to help them with the troubling problem of blood pressure care, and leading me to many hidden answers that have helped them, and many others, recover their health.

Gayle Eversole, September 2005
updated 2012

What is high blood pressure?

High blood pressure, or hypertension, means, according to medical information provided by a major drug company, high pressure (tension) in the arteries. It does not mean excess emotional stress, though stress from any source over a long period of time can contribute to high blood pressure.

• Blood pressure rises and falls with each heartbeat, even normal blood pressure does this. These levels can change with food, everyday activity, during exercise or when you are asleep, and this is also normal. However, in some people, and as we get older, changes in blood pressure start to happen at higher pressure levels than normal and this is what high blood pressure means. Some people do have a tendency to have higher than average blood pressure because of hereditary or intrinsic physiologic factors. Blood pressure is usually measured with a blood pressure cuff placed around the upper arm that registers the pressure in units called millimetres of mercury (or mm Hg).

• Blood pressure is usually considered to be high when it is at a level exceeding 140/90 mm Hg ("140 over 90") on several readings under various conditions. However, defining normal and abnormal is not always so clear-cut and your doctor or health care professional will take the necessary recommendations. New guidelines have lowered the definition by five or more points.

• Blood pressure rises and falls with each heartbeat.

Systolic blood pressure, the higher number, represents the pressure moving blood into your arteries and the circulation.

Diastolic pressure, the lower number, occurs as the heart relaxes following a beat. It represents the lowest pressure to which the arteries are exposed between heartbeats.

How do you get high blood pressure?

No specific cause is found in 95% of patients with hypertension. This is called primary hypertension or essential hypertension.

• Most people have primary or essential hypertension.

• Most cases of primary hypertension are because of increased stiffness and narrowing of the smaller (peripheral) arteries.

This causes increased resistance to the flow of blood and is what makes your blood pressure go up. Increased peripheral artery resistance is associated with genetics (family history), obesity, lack of exercise, over use of processed salt and the natural aging process.

• A few patients have high blood pressure with a known cause (secondary hypertension). Long-lasting (chronic) kidney disease accounts for most of these cases where there is excessive fluid accumulation in the body that raises blood pressure. We offer effective kidney cleansing products at Creating Health Institute.

• Hypertension can also occur during some pregnancies, often related to low magnesium and vitamin B levels.

How serious is high blood pressure?

It is rare these days for blood pressure to be so high as to pose an immediate threat to life. In almost all cases, the problem with blood pressure is that over time it can cause damage to the tiny blood vessels and this may affect the function of the heart, eyes and kidneys.

Again, over time it can affect the larger arteries as well and contribute to hardening of the arteries. This explains why people with untreated high blood pressure have a higher risk of suffering from a stroke, heart attack, heart failure, hardening of the arteries, and eye, glandular, or kidney problems.

For this reason medical treatment with a blood pressure lowering medicine is given for a long period of time, which in most cases is for life.

Because blood pressure tends to increase as you get older, it means blood pressure should be checked regularly, even if it is 'normal'.

How long does high blood pressure last?

High blood pressure may be present for several years before it is detected and is often found during a routine check-up. Usually there are no symptoms. Consequences may only become apparent after many years.

How is high blood pressure treated?

Doctors know that there is a benefit from treating high blood pressure at any age, even in older patients of 65 years and over. Depending on the blood pressure level different things are recommended. In some people with only mild elevations in blood pressure a change in diet and adopting a healthier lifestyle may reduce the blood pressure to normal.

A nutritional therapist or other natural health care practitioner can help you develop a healthy nutritional plan; it is more than getting rid of excess fluid or reducing the amount of salt you eat. There are other things you can change in your diet that can help. If you are overweight, weight loss will help significantly.

High blood pressure is usually treated with a range of different medicine, including:

• Beta-blockers cause the heart to beat more slowly and less strongly. They work by blocking the action of nerves supplying the heart that release a chemical called noradrenaline. This helps to control the rhythm and force of heart muscle movement. They also block a hormone called adrenaline. Adrenaline is the emergency responder (fight or flight) in the human body.

• Diuretics work in the kidneys to make you pass urine more often and help to eliminate excess fluid.

• Calcium-channel blockers relax arterial blood vessels making them less narrow and lower resistance to blood flow, allowing blood to flow more easily. They work by preventing calcium from entering the muscles in blood vessels because calcium contributes to the narrowing of blood vessels.

• ACE inhibitors and angiotensin II antagonists generally relax the blood vessels. They do this by preventing a hormone called angiotensin II from working, either by preventing its production or blocking its action. Like other hormones, angiotensin II is an active chemical signal in the blood. It controls the function of many organs or systems including the narrowing of blood vessels and prevents the kidneys from eliminating excess fluid. Doctors believe that angiotensin II is involved as one of the causes of high blood pressure.

It is also important to follow any lifestyle instructions that your doctor has given to you, like trying to give up smoking, reducing your weight, doing more exercise and eating a healthy diet. When these and other risk factors are present together with high blood pressure, then this means there is even higher risk of serious disease. It is also important to continue taking any medications you have been given, even if you feel normal.

Being Well Naturally

The preceding is good basic information you should know about high blood pressure; it is a silent killer.

As a natural health practitioner and medically trained professional, it is my belief, along with others, that hypertension can be cured. A serious problem, however, is the lack of effective medical treatment because a number of factors are not included in the medical approach.

This booklet will attempt to address some of these concerns and provide well-researched and documented natural healing techniques for the prevention, treatment and resolution of hypertension.

In The Beginning

Sound diet and nutrition principles are the foundation of health. Health building starts at an early age. For an infant breastfeeding offers the best start. In situations where a mother is unable to nurse her baby, avoiding soy-based formula is critical. Soy products have been proven to alter thyroid function and growth. Thyroid health and blood pressure are connected.

From a natural health perspective refraining from feeding grains and fruits to infants is highly recommended.

Vegetables should be the first food, and these should not be introduced until the baby is at least 6 months of age. The Happy Home Baby Food Grinder™ is a great way to start your child eating healthy, home prepared organic vegetables. If you are not able to purchase organic foods you can purchase a copy of our Healthy Food Soak©.

Food allergy is an issue today often related to the high number of vaccinations often forced on infants and children; Food additives, preservatives and glutamates such as MSG (sold as Accent), BHT, BHA, artificial sweeteners and newer synthetic salt and sugar flavorings should be avoided. Grains often cause allergy, as do other foods. Allergy causes inflammation and this may lead to hardening of the cardiovascular system over time. Allergy is often related to an imbalance of magnesium, potassium, sodium and calcium in the body. Other minerals involved are aluminum (causes the liver to become congested), chromium, selenium and zinc. Identifying and resolving food and environmental allergies has been shown in research done in the 1970s - 80s to reduce blood pressure to the normal range. Low levels of vitamin B6 and other important B vitamins are related to the buildup of plaque in the arterial bed. This is common because of the overuse of highly processed foods such as cereals and baked goods. The development of diabetes is also related to vitamin and mineral deficiencies in food. CHI strongly supports the relationship of allergy to the development of hypertension.

• Fat - Fats are very important to health. We believe that hydrogenated fat, margarine, very low and non-fat diets do not promote health. Healthy fats include flax oil, unsalted or cultured butter, olive oil, palm oil and coconut oil. The absorption of some critical vitamins and minerals depends on fat. Hormone health requires fat, as does the health of the brain and nervous system and cell wall membranes. Use healthy fats in moderation.

• Sugar - Sugars found in fruit and fruit juices can lead to the development sugar sensitivity and insulin resistance through over use and over exposure. Avoid using sugary drinks or foods and highly processed bakery items to prevent the development of digestive problems with sugar and non-complex carbohydrates.

Insulin resistance can be related to the development of hypertension and diabetes. Excessive sugar intake also plays a role in lowered immunity. Sugar and hydrogenated fat, in combination, can be very harmful to your health. Fructose and high-fructose corn syrup both stress the pancreas. We strongly encourage total avoidance of any artificial sweetener. Honey is an energizer and very nutritious. Use only local, raw, unpasteurized honey. Try our unique Low Heat Coconut Sugar, Xylitol, or unadulterated Stevia extract powder that is a good herbal sweetener safe for people with diabetes.

• Salt - Salt is a necessary ingredient for health. Some research shows that it is perhaps chloride that is more important, however sodium is needed too. Highly refined salt has all of the naturally occurring minerals cooked out of it to make it free flowing. Often additives are mixed with processed salt, including maltodextrin (a sugar) and fluoride.

Highly processed foods, especially diet, packaged cold cereals, prepared and fast foods contain high amounts of processed salt. Read labels to help you make good buying decisions about these food products. Since salt is necessary for life we suggest the use of Celtic salt or Blackfoot Traditional Salt®. These are unprocessed farmed and mined natural salts that have not shown a negative effect on health.

We do not recommend Himalayan salt because of high fluoride and other toxic metal levels.

Taoist Bamboo Salt is a highly purified living salt that is very helpful in the treatment of disease, including high blood pressure.

Learn more about salt in the work of John Laragh, MD.

• Water - Water is necessary for life. Many health problems can be improved by drinking about 3 litres of pure water daily. An easy way to accomplish this is to purchase good quality bottled water in the size that is just about a litre, or use distilled water. A litre is close in amount to a quart. Drink one bottle in the morning, one in the afternoon, and one in the evening. It is best to drink water about one-half hour before or after meals.

Very cold or ice water stresses digestion, and drinking too much water or other liquids during meals dilutes necessary digestive enzymes. Natural salt helps water do its work of cleansing and lubricating in the body.

• pH - pH is a measure of acid forming substances in your body. Balancing it is important to health. For many people with toxic systems more alkaline creating foods are suggested because imbalances can promote hypertension, inflammation or allergies. Apple Cider vinegar tea helps balance your pH and aids digestion. Healthy pH, measured in saliva should be slightly below 7, ideally 6.4. It is best to measure this at 2 pm daily.

We encourage organic food. Behind our strong belief in favor of non-GMO organic food is quality, enhanced availability of vitamins and minerals, and improved nutritional status.

Chemical herbicides and pesticides generally are not used in organic farming.

Environmental toxins do build up in the body; residues are stored in fat, and they can be disease producing. These toxins are a contributing factor to lowered immune status. The Leaflady's Brown Rice cleanse is a good way to help use food to remove heavy metals and other toxins.

Avoid smoking and smog. Alteration of the oxygen content in blood by pollutants has a negative effect on the body.

Creating Health Institute (CHI) in conjunction with The Oake Centre for natural health education and Health Forensics, offers educational programs, counseling and nutritional support to help you stop smoking, other health concerns and with supplements, water and air purification systems.

Vitamin B15, DMG, Mag Phos and Ferrum Phos Cell Salts aid the promotion of oxygen in the body. Follow label directions.

Reduce or eliminate caffeine from your diet. Caffeine reduces magnesium, can irritate the kidneys and bladder, and stresses the liver and adrenal glands.

Vitamin D shows good support too. It has been found effective in lowering plasma renin and angiotensin II levels and lowering blood pressure. The bio active form is D3.

Use enzymes with your meals. Protease enzymes dramatically improve chronically obstructed arteries.

Numerous cross-over, single-blind and placebo studies have confirmed this. Intravenous therapy with plant protease is dramatically more effective than anti-coagulant therapy (heparin, warfarin) at re-canalizing obstructed arteries and improving blood flow through obstructed arterial segments. We also encourage probiotics.

Reduce or eliminate excessive alcohol consumption. It is known, however, that small amounts of red wine can benefit health.

Grapes, especially red, blue, and black grapes have more anti-oxidants. The seeds are an exceptionally good source of phytonutrients called pycnogenol and proanthocyanidins. The skins are a source of resveratrol, and anti-aging compounds that help with many health concerns, including blood pressure. Balsamic vinegar is made from the remains of grape pressing, including skins and seeds.

Exercise for the body and the mind will serve you and your health well over the years.

Exercise is a good start to prevent the current trend of obesity in very young children and others of all ages. These programs should include proper deep breathing exercises.

So you see building a healthy foundation for your body is just like building a strong foundation for your home.

What we think about drugs

Dr. Allen Roses, vice-president of genetics for GlaxoSmithKline, openly stated that "...more than 90% of drugs work in 30% to 50% of the people."

Patients and physicians have learned that treating hypertension with drugs is "hit or miss" and drug changes are common. Using drugs in combination may cause true functional health problems. Hypertension therapy today is based on drugs that have side effects that may be incapacitating for some people.

Properly prescribed pharmaceutical drugs cause 100,000 to 350,000 deaths annually in hospitals and medical practice according to the American Medical Association. Overall, prescription drugs are now known to be the major leading cause of death in mainstream medicine. When drugs are prescribed for a health problem, it is usually only symptoms that are treated.

Health Forensics offers a unique service to help you properly evaluate your prescribed medications in an effort to reduce any problems you may encounter.

Hypertension is a symptom of something going on inside the body. If it is arterial resistance then looking at ways to improve vascular health is an option. If the symptom is water retention enhancing kidney function or increasing highly digestible protein in the diet may be of help.

The idea is to ask your doctor what might be going on and become a better advocate for your own good health. Drugs have serious side effects. Often you might not know what these are even though there is a legal requirement to provide you with this information before prescribing a drug.

Do not stop taking any prescribed medication without consulting the prescribing physician.

Beta-Blockers can have an effect on thyroid function and thereby lead to the development of hypertension and increased blood pressure if you are prescribed this medication.

Diuretics can cause loss of potassium, an important heart mineral. Often doctors prescribe potassium supplements along with diuretics. Over time mineral losses can lead to osteoporosis when using diuretics.

One of the most commonly prescribed diuretics is Lasix or furosemide. Lasix was developed for short-term or intermittent use. Long term use of this type of diuretic, which has become more common over the years, can lead to increased doses to accomplish the job because of ineffectiveness.

Calcium channel blockers can cause sudden death. These are interesting drugs because they lower your heart rate substantially. This may cause problems in peripheral circulation because blood is not getting pumped into critical organs or feet and toes. Calcium is necessary for heart function and blood pressure maintenance. If these functions are blocked by a drug you might develop other problems.

Aspirin is often used in conjunction with drugs. Aspirin can cause silent bleeding and clotting disorders. Also, daily aspirin may lead to the development of pancreatic cancer.

Aspirin should not be taken with certain calcium channel blockers such as Norvasc. Daily aspirin treatment can lead to thyroid imbalance (low) and create increased pain perception pathways.

ACE inhibitors cause problems too, but interestingly, before these drugs were in wide use, magnesium was used to accomplish the same result. Yes, magnesium is nature's ACE inhibitor. Emergency doctors up on the research are returning to the use of this heart healthy mineral.

Statins
I do not endorse cholesterol lowering drugs used in the medical treatment of hypertension. These drugs have serious risks for liver and heart failure, and may promote cancer and hepatitis C. Statins can also cause rhabdomyolysis, causing muscle cramping from cell breakdown, which may lead to kidney failure. Red Rice Yeast is a statin and may cause some of these same problems.

Refer to the work of Uffe Ravnskov, MD, PhD for more data on the cholesterol myth.

Necessary nutrients for heart health blocked by the statin drugs include Co-enzyme Q10, vitamins A-D-E and several B complex vitamins.

Low thyroid function often leads to increased cholesterol (LDL) and triglyceride levels. Make sure you get thorough and proper diagnostic testing for these concerns.

Now For the Natural

First, of course, communicate with your health care provider. Secondly do work to improve your diet and lifestyle.

Following on the basics, here are some of the things that I have used with our clients.

I've included effective methods from other doctors and natural practitioners too.

Remember that Harvard Medical School showed, in a 1997 study, that diet can reduce blood pressure as much as drugs.

Food

• Apple Cider vinegar drink is a helpful beverage to provide potassium and reduce cholesterol and plaque buildup. Use organic, raw and unfiltered ACV. Take 1 to 2 teaspoons in a glass of water before meals. The many benefits of ACV for health were established in the writing of D.C. Jarvis, MD. The use of vinegar for health dates back to Hippocrates in 425 BC.

• Applesauce and plain yoghurt - this blend helps the arterial vessels remain pliable. Mix 1/3 cup organic or homemade applesauce and 1/3 cup plain, organic low-fat or whole milk homemade yoghurt. Homemade yoghurt is very easy to make and has many health promoting benefits. To learn how to make your own yoghurt, please contact CHI for our recipe.

• Beets are helpful for the liver, aid digestion and help remove fat from the liver. Beets are a source of Nitric oxide. I've written a lengthy article on beets in an issue of my newsletter, *hebalYODA Says!*

• Celery and pineapple are foods that help lower blood pressure. Carrots help reduce the risk of stroke.

• Dexter Morris, M.D. (University of North Carolina) says that phytochemicals keep your heart healthy. Chlorophyll is a major phytochemical anti-oxidant and it neutralizes aflatoxins from mold. CHI's offers organic chlorophyll rich products.

• Foods high in potassium include oranges, potatoes, squash, apricots, lima beans, bananas, avocado, tomato, and peaches.

• Fish Oil and other Essential Fatty Acids (EFA) help prevent cellular aggregation. These food sources provide important fat-soluble vitamins needed for health, and help keep cell wall membrane pliable and strong. High GLA oils may help lower blood pressure and improve circulation. Try Borage oil or Evening Primrose oil or a blend with Flax oil (women only) or Extra Virgin Olive oil.

• Fiber, and the wonderful health foods apple and oats, reduces problems of constipation and related hypertension.

High quality probiotics provide beneficial bacteria to help with this, as does goat whey. Remember that vegetables are high in fiber.

• Have adequate, but moderate, amounts of protein in your diet to support health and cell repair.

• Onions contain allergy fighting chemicals, including quercetin and prostaglandin A1 that act like a hormone to lower blood pressure.

• Parsley, a very effective diuretic herb is high in potassium. A handful makes a refreshing tea.

• Tomatoes have lycopene, an antioxidant that may be as effective as vitamin E.

• Reishi Mushroom contains several chemical constituents including sterols, coumarin, mannitol, polysaccharides, and triterpenoids called ganoderic acids. Ganoderic acids may lower blood pressure as well as decrease low density lipoprotein (LDL) and triglyceride levels. These specific triterpenoids also help reduce blood platelets from sticking together - an important factor in lowering the risk for coronary artery disease.

• Walnuts, ¼ cup daily, supply beneficial support to the heart in the form of essential fatty acids and vitamin E. Avoid any GMO oils especially soy, canola, or corn that are touted as a source of vitamin E.

According to the University of California, Berkeley, studies have shown that nuts can help prevent coronary disease. They're rich in unsaturated fats, vitamin E, fiber, folic acid (B9), and other B vitamins. Eat them raw, after soaking overnight in pure water to make the nutrients more absorbable. Raw almonds supply magnesium and calcium. Store all raw nuts in the freezer to avoid rancidity.

• Watermelon - Watermelon and watermelon seed tea are well-known and very effective diuretics. This food also helps cleanse the kidneys.

• Wheat Germ Oil – The famous vitamin E studies done in the 1950s by the Schute brothers (both were MDs) in Canada used wheat germ oil as the source of vitamin E. If using other types of remedies use the mixed tocopherols and avoid the synthetic forms of vitamin E (d-l tocopherol) which is only half as effective as the natural form (d).

Tocotrienols are more expensive but show good effect and also help with cholesterol. Vitamin E will prevent platelet agglutination (sticky cells) and act as a "thinner". Vitamin E also insures that oxygen is carried to vital organs such as the heart. Vitamin E will help prevent certain debilitation for people with diabetes that are associated with circulation and peripheral neuropathy.

Foods high in magnesium, potassium and calcium may help prevent and lower high blood pressure. Ask about our nutrition counseling and resources.

Herbs

• Cayenne – High in vitamin C, helps other herbs, reduces arterial plaque.

• Dandelion and Milk Thistle promote liver health. Dandelion will also benefit the kidneys. We also suggest our Kidney Rescue Formula for healthy kidneys.

• Hawthorn, the heart herb - Improves heart function, heart valve strength and electrical conductivity. Hawthorn combines well with the nervous system calming herb Motherwort.

• Herbal Chelation – This oral treatment helps cleanse the interior of blood vessels and makes them more pliable. It removes heavy metals. Other chelation therapies include the use of intravenous EDTA. EDTA has been controversial but many integrative physicians realize its benefits. Medical providers of this treatment are listed with the Association of Oxidative Medicine.

• Instead of Aspirin – Ginger (anti-inflammatory and a digestive aid), Red Clover Blossom (contains naturally occurring coumadin and helps "thick blood"), White Willow Bark (nature's aspirin), or Gingko ("blood thinner").

• Other heart helping herbs – mistletoe (tones the heart without resorting to the use of digitalis) and lily-of-the-valley have cardiotonic and diuretic effects; valerian root (relaxes muscles, arterioles and the arterial system); wild cherry bark (works on the pituitary to affect hormonal balancing); goldenseal (*an endangered herb, burns up triglygerides and lowers blood sugar); silica (strengthens the arterial walls).

• Siberian Ginseng – Supports the adrenal glands that play an active role in hormonal influence of fluid balance and blood pressure.

• Wild Bear's Garlic – Russian scientific studies show that garlic is one of the two specific natural substances effective in the treatment of hypertension (Buckwheat, high in rutin, is the second). The tops of this species of garlic are used for heart health and they contain three times the ACE inhibitory effect of regular garlic. This species contains higher levels of ajoenes, adenosine, iron, and ACE-Inhibitory potential. In fact, it has the highest natural sulfur and adenosine levels found anywhere in the plant kingdom! Adenosine is a key component in the regulation of hypertension and tachycardia. Wild Bear's Garlic has circulation increasing and lipid-reducing properties that may be useful help in preventing heart attacks. I also use a unique high potency water extract of garlic – 36 cloves per capsule.

New studies show that garlic, ginger and selenium are very effective for reducing inflammation and offer significant anti aging benefit.

• Other helping herbs are linden (blossom), wood betony (leaves, flowers), yarrow (leaves, flowers), lavender, olive leaf and cactus grandiflorus.

Vitamins and Minerals

• Vitamin B 12 shots – a treatment you will have to get from your doctor, is effective for treating hypertension in women only. Contact CHI for this protocol, proven over decades in orthomolecular (nutritional) medicine.

• High absorption magnesium - Magnesium is nature's ACE inhibitor. This mineral is often found to be low in tissue samples of patients with hypertension. Adding magnesium (Mg.) rich foods to your diet or using our favorite supplements (Mg. Lactate or Mg. Malate) may be helpful.

• Vitamin C and Bioflavonoids - Vitamin C is a chelator and highly effective in reversing atherosclerosis. Bioflavonoids are synergistic parts of the vitamin C complex, often including rutin and hesperidin. It is also nature's perfect statin: see the study titled "Inhibition of HMG-CoA reductase activity by ascorbic acid" at http://www.jbc.org/cgi/content/abstract/261/16/7127.

Frederick Klenner, MD wrote: "Some physicians would stand by and see their patient die rather than use ascorbic acid (Vitamin C) because in their finite minds it exists only as a vitamin." Vitamin C is remarkably safe even in enormously high doses. Compared to commonly used prescription drugs, side effects are virtually nonexistent. It does not cause kidney stones. In fact, Vitamin C increases urine flow and favorably lowers the pH to help keep stones from forming.

William J. McCormick, MD used Vitamin C since the late 1940's to prevent and treat kidney stones. Vitamin C does not significantly raise oxalate levels, and uric acid stones have never resulted from its use. Dr. Klenner said, "The ascorbic acid/ kidney stone story is a myth." These parts of the vitamin C complex act as free radical scavengers.

• Vitamin D is now showing very good results in lowering blood pressure. You need limited exposure to the sun, without sunscreen, to help your body make this necessary vitamin. Low vitamin D levels may be a key factor in the greater incidence of hypertension in people of color, because dark skin is slow to absorb vitamin D. This is true also for the elderly and those who avoid the sun, or may be institutionalized. Use D3 for best results.

• Amino Acids - Arginine has been shown to be somewhat effective in certain studies for increasing heart cell health and strength, and improving ventricular pumping. Taurine, Cysteine, Methionine, Proline and Lysine may also have good benefit.

• B complex vitamins – These very important vitamins are necessary for heart health and offer many protective supportive functions in your body. A good source of B complex vitamins is nutritional yeast. Mix 1 - 2 tablespoons daily in sour juice (grapefruit) to avoid the gas if you are not accustomed to high nutrient density foods. Vitamin B3 or niacin can be used to lower cholesterol and triglycerides. B6, B12 and Folic Acid (B9) are known to reduce homocysteine levels. Take a complete B complex as a foundation when taking single B vitamins. This helps avoid loss of effectiveness of these heart healthy vitamins and the possibility of neuropathy.

• Choline (part of the B vitamin family found in Lecithin) Lecithin lowers cholesterol and acts to help keep your brain and nervous system healthy. It also keeps cell wall membranes pliable. Inositol is usually paired with this.

• COQ10 – This important co-enzyme is especially necessary for a healthy heart. It oxygenates the fuel cells (mitochondria) of the body. COQ10 is depleted by cholesterol lowering drugs. CoQ10 is best taken with healthy fatty foods, vitamin E or olive oil. Take 100 mg. to 300 mg. daily.

• Potassium – Gayelord Hauser's Vegetable (potassium) Broth (see suggested foods above). Use as a broth or add to food and salad dressing. Potassium helps carry insulin across the cell wall membrane. Alfalfa provides potassium, other vitamins and minerals, chlorophyll and protein.

• Minerals benefit health. Use a quality trace mineral and multi-vitamin product daily.

• Whole grain raw cereal (Muesli) – Dr. Johann Georg Schnitzer, MD, from Germany, uses this old natural (Natur Doktor) remedy. You may know it as Familia, or Grizzlies' Organic Raw Muesli. This is a whole grain cereal ground just before preparation in the morning. It is "cooked" with hot water by steeping, then eaten with raw apple and chopped almonds that have been soaked overnight. He decries the protein excess of Western countries as a major factor in hypertension.

Dr. Schnitzer states "English speaking populations don't expect that there is any cure, so they don't even get the idea to search for a cure. German speaking people search for "Bluthochdruck heilen" (= hypertension cure)."
http://www.dr-schnitzer.de/hypertensionstudy02-introduction.html

Other Helps

• Acupuncture and Electro-Acupuncture – consult with a well-trained and experienced acupuncturist.

• Address causes of emotionally related hypertension – work with a counselor or therapist you can trust. The Spiritual side of heart health relates to unresolved, longstanding emotional problems. Joyously release the past and be at peace.

• Aromatherapy - Ylang Ylang is a pure essential oil effective for hypertension. Sniff some on a tissue or make a spray bottle for your room and office.

• Biofeedback - This is one of the methods used by Herbert Benson, MD (Type A personality) in studies done at Harvard Medical School decades ago. AFT, or Attractor Field Therapy, is another similar treatment you can do at home. See http://www.the-tree-of-life.com

• Chiropractic – certain forms of chiropractic are effective for lowering blood pressure. Avoid the high force techniques.

Try resonance equipment.

• Deep Breathing - Slow deep breathing or Yoga or square breathing is well documented for relaxation and lowering blood pressure.

• Eat small, frequent meals and occasionally under eat. Most natural health practitioners suggest resting digestion once a week to help with this. Order Leaflady's Rejuvenation Cleansing Fast to help with this.

• Energetic remedies for cardiovascular health from DNR have helped many people since 1894 recover their health. http://www.dnrsite.com/store4.mv? AFFIL=9481408

• Exercise – Rebounding, Walking, Yoga, or Tai Chi: These are effective exercise techniques that help you strengthen your body, build collateral circulation and improve general health and well-being. Muscle strengthening exercise is beneficial. You can get good help from physical therapy or a qualified trainer.

• Homeopathy – this very effective technique, scientifically proven to be effective.

Flower Essence Therapy are examples of good therapies for emotional cause of disease.

These therapies will affect physical conditions with resolution of underlying issues. For example, Homeopathic Aluminum helps reduce aluminum buildup from liver stores that may lead to lower blood pressure.

• Massage - Relaxes muscles and helps remove toxins from the body. Far Infrared Sauna can help improve the benefit of massage.

• Reflexology, a special massage technique of the feet, hands, or ears has reduced blood pressure effectively. Cobblestone mats and acupressure sandals can help. See http://www.reflexology-research.com/jan2004reflexions.html

• Meditation – Has a similar affect to Biofeedback.

• Reiki and other energy healing. Ask for our Introductory Guide, available with a donation to Creating Health Institute.

• Use Leaflady's liver cleansing recipe periodically to help reduce the toxic load in the liver and blood. See Liver Help file – http://leaflady.org/fasting.htm.

Low Blood Pressure

Low Blood Pressure is often considered to be a health condition in which there is a diminished ability in the body to respond to fluctuations in pressure changes in the cardiovascular system. Most often this is called orthostatic hypotension. Most people experience this on standing or rising from a lying position like getting out of bed in the morning. Many times low blood pressure is ignored by physicians. It is generally defined as blood pressure below the normal range (120/80 is the standard normal for adults, 115/75 is the new range). Medical treatment is based on the cause.

There are a number of causes of this condition:

• Drugs that interferes with the autonomic nervous system

• Diseases that interfere with the autonomic nervous system

• Lack of blood volume because of blood loss or anemia

• Weak adrenal and thyroid or other endocrine function

• Vitamin and mineral deficiencies

• Idiopathic (no cause found)

Symptoms may include fainting, seizures, blurred vision, weakness, and light-headedness. Overlooked warning signs of low blood pressure may include diabetes, kidney disease, pernicious anemia and Parkinson's disease, porphyria or Guillain-Barré syndrome.

Treatment should be focused on the cause, and proper evaluation is necessary, as hypotension in certain cases can be serious, and even life-threatening.

Tests may include blood work, glandular function testing, review of current medications, Hair Mineral Analysis (HTMA) and metabolic testing for imbalances. Many tests, including HTMA, may be ordered through CHI.

Natural treatment may include:

• Zinc
• B complex, select B vitamins and nutritional yeast

- Thiamine (vitamin B1)
- Vitamin E and K
- Vitamin C and Bioflavonoids
- Raw Adrenal Concentrate
- Potassium supplementation
- Sodium supplementation
- Phosphorus supplementation
- Pantothenic Acid (vitamin B5)
- Magnesium chelates
- Licorice root tea or tincture
- Siberian Ginseng
- DHEA (avoid unless you have been tested for DHEA
levels)
- Astragalus – we suggest Herbal Fortress™ brand
- Evening Primrose, Borage or Black Currant oil
- Iodine or adding seaweed (know your source) to your diet.
- Homeopathic cell salts

Foods and Fasting

A wholesome diet is very important. Early naturopaths, practicing when food was available without the additives and processing of today, often recommended:

• Homemade cottage cheese, milk, butter and cheese.
• Whole grains, raw nuts and seeds.
• Peas, potatoes and steamed broccoli
• Calve's Liver or liver capsules.

Some recommend eating red meat in small amounts of about one and one-half ounces weekly. Beef in Oriental Medicine is considered a neutral food to stimulate liver function.

People with hypotension may fast, but this should be done in conjunction with a knowledgeable health care provider.

Helpful juices include pineapple, celery, black radish, parsley, carrot, red beet, grapes, onion and garlic.

Traditionally cayenne, dandelion, garlic, ginger and kelp have helped strengthen the circulatory system.

These herbs also assist in balancing blood pressure levels. Find kelp and other good foods in our Naturally Nutritional Seasoning.

Herbal iron support is helpful when anemia is present. Nettle herb is used traditionally for anemia.

Lemon water and pure essential oil of lemon may help strengthen the nervous system through its action on the parasympathetic nervous system. It helps strengthen and stimulate smooth muscle and raises blood pressure through action via the anterior and posterior lobes of the hypothalamus. Some aroma-therapists associate lemon essential oil with lowering blood pressure.

Rosemary essential oil is generally used for hypertension because it stimulates blood circulation. It may help hypotension because of its action on the heart.

Rosemary should be used with care if you have experienced seizures. As with most essential oils, avoid use during pregnancy.

Avoid canned, refined and high cholesterol foods, caffeine, all artificial sweeteners and flavoring.

Other Helps:

• Acupressure, Acupuncture and Electro-Acupuncture

• Chiropractic or Osteopathic manipulation

• Deep Breathing exercises to oxygenate the blood and internal organs

• Hot and Cold Alternating Foot Baths

• Meditation

• Reflexology

• Dry Skin Brushing improves circulation and lymph drainage (both high and low blood pressure and skin health).

The Erdman Clinic in Havertown, Pennsylvania used a therapy developed by Dr. Erdman, a specialist in physical medicine. This treatment used the application of cold to locations along the spinal column. It was a very effective treatment, and helped thousands who suffered with low blood pressure. The clinic remains open today; however, the Erdman Method may no longer be practiced, following the doctor's death. Books may be available.

Emotional and Spiritual Considerations

Louis Hay defines low blood pressure as "defeatism and lack of love as a child".

Her affirmation for this condition is: "My life is a joy! I NOW choose to live in the ever-joyous now."

Healing

Healing occurs on four levels: physical, mental, emotional and spiritual. Without the inclusion of all four levels in your healing program, you may not achieve your goal. Most often the spiritual is forgotten.

Appendix

Quick Guide to Using Herbal Remedies

To get the maximum benefit from herbal remedies they must be properly prepared. Women of childbearing age should always make sure the herbs are safe for use during pregnancy.

Infusions - An infusion is prepared by adding 1 to 2 teaspoons of dried herb (or 2 to 4 teaspoons of fresh herb) to 8-10 ounces of freshly boiled pure water, and steep for 10-15 minutes before straining. It's best to use a ceramic pot with a lid, or glass canning jar.

The standard dosage is one cup three times a day. It may be taken hot or cold. Infusions prepared for colds and flu should be taken hot. Strong infusions are made by adding the herbs to about a pint of water and allowing to steep overnight, strain and drink throughout the next day. Herbal teas are considered infusions.

Decoctions – These are teas made with bark and twigs and seeds brought gently to a boil, and then reduced to low heat.

Keeping covered, simmer for about 10-20 minutes, then strain. Use 1 to 2 teaspoons of herb per cup of cold water.

The usual dosage is 1 cup three times a day. If the herb is very bitter or strong, use 4 teaspoons three times a day.

Prepare no more than 24 hours in advance.

Tincture - A tincture is an alcoholic extraction of herb.

Alcohol dissolves the active constituents out of the plant matter and acts as a preservative. Vinegar or vegetable glycerin may also be used. Any part of the plant may be used.

Place 4 ounces of dried herb in a glass jar with a tight-fitting lid and add 2 cups 100 proof vodka. Some use 20% water and 80% vodka. Let this jar sit in a cupboard for two weeks, shaking daily. Then strain through an unbleached muslin cloth into a brown glass bottle. Keep tightly closed. The standard dosage is 15 or more drops three times daily, depending on the herbal tincture you are making, added to a small amount of water.

Dose is adjusted by weight, especially for use with children, small adults and Elders, using Clark's Rule (percentage of adult dose x weight of child).

I like to start tinctures on the new moon and strain on the full moon, according to the 'bio-natura' philosophy.

Capsules - Dry, powdered herb can be placed inside empty capsules. This method is preferred by some people who do tolerate the taste of bitter herbs. The average adult dose, based on a person weighing 150 pounds, is six capsules daily, taken in divided doses of 2 capsules, 3 times daily. It saves to make your capsules with a capsule maker, available from CHI.

Other methods of using herbs are syrups, oils, wines, creams, ointments, suppositories, compresses, inhalants, and a poultice or foment.

RESOURCES

As a health care professional, specializing in natural health care, I am here to help you, and it is one of the reasons that I compiled this book. I want people to have access to the same information I have learned in the many years of this fulfilling work.

Please contact us through our website, www.leaflady.org for more information on resources and the myriad of scientific and medical literature available that supports the information presented in this book. We realize that there are many skeptics in mainstream medicine; we just extend the challenge to them to do a thorough search of the literature. Please contact us with your questions, comments and requests for products or consultation. We offer discounts on consultations and products to those supporting our work through purchases of this publication.

All profits from the sale of this book go to support the community programs of Creating Health Institute (CHI), a 501c3 tax-exempt, non-profit organization. We welcome your thoughtful donations as well.

IMPORTANT READER INFORMATION

The material presented here is not complete nor is it prescriptive. It is for educational purposes only. None of the information is to be construed as medical advice. It serves only as a guide to assist you and your health care provider in selecting options to help you best address your concerns with blood pressure care. Before applying any therapy or use of herbs and nutritional supplements, you may want to seek advice from your health care provider.

Information presented in this publication should not be interpreted as a substitute for physician evaluation or treatment by a health care professional.

***Wishing you joy
and the best for your health and healing!***

About the Author

Gayle Eversole, DHom, PhD, MH, NP, ND, has been studying and using natural healing for more than 50 years. She received her nursing degree from Neumann College in Aston, PA, and is a member of Sigma Theta Tau, national honor society for nursing there. She has worked for more than thirty five years in the medical profession as a nurse practitioner, consultant, administrator and educator. She serves on the medical advisory board of several health organizations and has worked in health care planning. Dr. Eversole offers legal and forensic nursing and mediation /arbitration for health concerns and Indian health issues, and is a widely respected health coach. She serves as a consultant to nutrition and herbal product companies, hosts a radio program, publishes a natural health eZINE, and maintains a clinical practice specializing in complex and complicated health problems. She is the author of My Happy Garden and My Medicine Garden and contributes to many books and articles on natural health care. Dr. Eversole continues to do research in natural health care, enjoys public speaking and writing articles in this field.

She has two grown daughters, one an artist working in the healing arts and one working in public relations.

Dr. Eversole offers classes to health care professionals, members of the public, business, organizations and government agencies.

For more information please see Health Forensics, www.healthforensics.org.

www.ingramcontent.com/pod-product-compliance
Lightning Source LLC
Chambersburg PA
CBHW020329290526
45785CB00007B/2969